"You matter because you are yc … we can not only to help
you die peacefully, but also to li … s, the founder of the
modern Hospice Movement, re … es offer to the dying and
to their loved ones at a very cha … . We are also mindful in
these days of the continued con … can offer to the ongoing
public discourse around the ethi … moral questions of Assisted Dying.

I am, therefore, most grateful to Father Michael Stack for this timely reflection on the importance and place of the Hospice and for offering his own considerable experience and insights of caring for the dying through his own ministry as a Hospice Chaplain.

Father Michael reminds us that many women and men have dedicated their lives over the centuries to the unique ministry of care for the sick and dying. Many remain unaware of the doctors, nurses, chaplains, volunteers, and carers who specialise in this particular area and who accompany those receiving end-of-life care. With over 200 Hospices for adults and 50 for children in England and Wales it is worth remembering that this care remains free for all.

Father Michael shares 10 accounts of patients he has accompanied through the course of his ministry and who have received this end-of-life care. He also reminds us that we may not always be aware of the location of our nearest Hospice, but Staff at all Hospices are always welcoming and open to answer any questions people may have.

As well as a tribute to Dame Cicely Saunders, as the modern-day founder of the Hospice Movement, Father Michael also acknowledges the work of Monica Pierce and Marie Hessian, who together with the help of Archbishop George Patrick Dwyer, the Archbishop of Birmingham in 1979, established the St Mary's Hospice at Selly Park in Birmingham. Following a merger in 2021 with the John Taylor Hospice at Erdington in Birmingham, it has now been renamed the Birmingham Hospice.

I wish to thank Father Michael Stack for this important and inspirational work, which also reflects the care and dedication of so many who work within the hospice setting and to whom I offer the assurance of my prayers and deepest gratitude.

✠ Bernard Longley

Archbishop of Birmingham

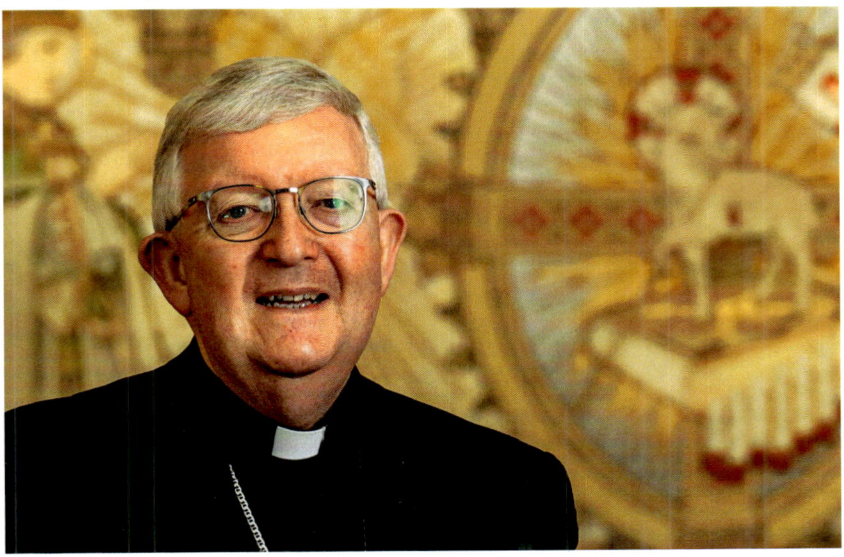

Extracts from the message of Pope Francis for the Feast of Our Lady of Lourdes, World Day of the Sick – February 11th 2023

Illness is part of our human condition. Yet, if illness is experienced in isolation and abandonment, unaccompanied by care and compassion, it can become inhumane.

When we go on a journey with others, it is not unusual for someone to feel sick, to have to stop because of fatigue or of some mishap along the way. It is precisely in such moments that we see *how* we are walking together: whether we are truly companions on the journey, or merely individuals on the same path, looking after our own interests and leaving others to "make do". For this reason, on the thirty-first World Day of the Sick, as the whole Church journeys along the synodal path, I invite all of us to reflect on the fact that it is especially through the experience of vulnerability and illness that we can learn to walk together according to the style of God, which is closeness, compassion, and tenderness.

In the Book of the Prophet Ezekiel, the Lord speaks these words that represent one of the high points of God's Revelation: "I myself will be the shepherd of my sheep, and I will make them lie down, says the Lord God.. I will seek the lost, and I will bring back the strayed, and I will bind up the injured, and I will strengthen the weak [...] I will feed them with justice" (34:15-16). Experiences of bewilderment, sickness, and weakness are part of the human journey. Far from excluding us from God's people, they bring us to the centre of the Lord's attention, for he is our Father and does not want to lose even one of his children along the way. Let us learn from him, then, how to be a community that truly walks together, capable of resisting the throwaway culture.

The Encyclical *Fratelli Tutti* encourages us to read anew the parable of the Good Samaritan, which I chose in order to illustrate how we can move from the "dark clouds" of a closed world to "envisaging and engendering an open world" (cf. No. 56). There is a profound link between this parable of Jesus and the many ways in which fraternity is denied in today's world. In particular, the fact that the man, beaten and robbed, is *abandoned* on the side of the road represents the condition in which all too many of our brothers and sisters are left at a time when they most need help. It is no longer easy to distinguish the assaults on human life and dignity that arise from natural causes from those caused by injustice and violence. In fact, increasing levels of inequality and the prevailing interests of the few now affect every human environment to the extent that it is difficult to consider any experience as having solely "natural" causes. All suffering takes place in the context of a "culture" and its various contradictions.

Here it is especially important to recognize the condition of loneliness and abandonment. This kind of cruelty can be overcome more easily than any other injustice, because – as the parable tells us – it only takes a moment of our attention, of being moved to compassion within us, in order to eliminate it. Two travellers, considered pious and religious, see the wounded man, yet fail to stop. The third passer-by, however, a Samaritan, a scorned foreigner, is moved with compassion and takes care of that stranger on the road, treating him as a brother. In doing so, without even thinking about it, he makes a difference, he makes the world more fraternal.

Brothers and sisters, we are rarely prepared for illness. Oftentimes, we fail even to admit that we are getting older. Our vulnerability frightens us and the pervasive culture of efficiency pushes us to sweep it under the carpet, leaving no room for our human frailty. In this way, when evil bursts onto the scene and wounds us, we are left stunned. Moreover, others might abandon us at such times. Or, in our own moments of weakness, we may feel that we should abandon others in order to avoid becoming a burden. This is how loneliness sets in, and we can become poisoned by a bitter sense of injustice, as if God himself had abandoned us. Indeed, we may find it hard to remain at peace with the Lord when our relationship with others and with ourselves is damaged. It is crucial, then, even in the midst of illness, that the whole Church measure herself against the Gospel example of the Good Samaritan, in order that she may become a true "field hospital", for her mission is manifested in acts of care, particularly in the historical circumstances of our time. We are all fragile and vulnerable, and need that compassion which knows how to pause, approach, heal, and raise up. Thus, the plight of the sick is a call that cuts through indifference and slows the pace of those who go on their way as if they had no sisters and brothers.

The World Day of the Sick calls for prayer and closeness towards those who suffer. Yet it also aims to raise the awareness of God's people, healthcare institutions and civil society with regard to a new way of moving forward together. The above-quoted prophecy of Ezekiel judges harshly the priorities of those who wield economic, cultural, and political power over others: "You eat the fat, you clothe yourselves with the wool, you slaughter the fatlings; but you do not feed the sheep. You have not strengthened the weak, you have not healed the sick, you have not bound up the injured, you have not brought back the strayed, you have not sought the lost, but with force and harshness you have ruled them" (34:3-4). God's word is always illuminating and timely; not only in what it denounces, but also in what it proposes. Indeed, the conclusion of the parable of the Good Samaritan suggests how the exercise of fraternity, which began as a face-to-face encounter, can be expanded into organized care. The elements of the inn, the innkeeper, the money and the promise to remain informed of the situation (cf. *Lk* 10:34-35) all point to the commitment of healthcare and social workers, family members and volunteers, through whom good stands up in the face of evil every day, in every part of the world.

These past years of the pandemic have increased our sense of gratitude for those who work each day in the fields of healthcare and research. Yet it is not enough to emerge from such an immense collective tragedy simply by honouring heroes. Covid-19 has strained the great networks of expertise and solidarity, and has exposed the structural limits of existing public welfare systems. Gratitude, then, needs to be matched by actively seeking, in every country, strategies and resources in order to guarantee each person's fundamental right to basic and decent healthcare.

The Samaritan calls the innkeeper to "take care of him" (*Lk* 10:35). Jesus addresses the same call to each of us. He exhorts us to "go and do likewise" (*Lk* 10:37). As I noted in *Fratelli Tutti*, "The parable shows us how a community can be rebuilt by men and women who identify with the vulnerability of others, who reject the creation of a society of exclusion, and act instead as neighbours, lifting up and rehabilitating the fallen for the sake of the common good" (No. 67). Indeed, "we were created for a fulfilment that can only be found in love. We cannot be indifferent to suffering" (No. 68).

On 11 February 2023, let us turn our thoughts to the Shrine of Lourdes, a prophetic lesson entrusted to the Church for our modern times. It is not only what functions well or those who are productive that matter. Sick people, in fact, are at the centre of God's people, and the Church advances together with them as a sign of a humanity in which everyone is precious and no one should be discarded or left behind.

To the intercession of Mary, Health of the Sick, I entrust all of you who are ill; you who care for them in your families, or through your work, research and volunteer service; and those of you who are committed to weaving personal, ecclesial, and civic bonds of fraternity. To all, I impart my heartfelt blessing."

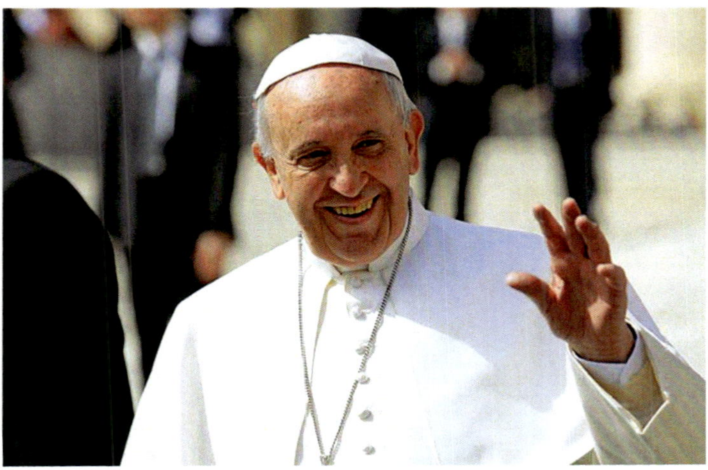

Pastoral Letter on Assisted Suicide 12/13 October 2024

My brothers and sisters,

This Wednesday, 16 October 2024, a bill will be introduced to Parliament proposing a change in the law to permit assisted suicide. The debate will continue for a number of months, in society and in Parliament, before a definitive vote is held there. This puts in the spotlight crucial questions about the dignity of human life and the care and protection afforded by our society to every human being.

As this debate unfolds there are three points I would like to put before you. I hope that you will take part in the debate, whenever and wherever you can, and that you will write to your Member of Parliament.

The first point is this: Be careful what you wish for.

No doubt the bill put before Parliament will be carefully framed, providing clear and very limited circumstances in which it would become lawful to assist, directly and deliberately, in the ending of a person's life. But please remember, the evidence from every single country in which such a law has been passed is clear: that the circumstances in which the taking of a life is permitted are widened and widened, making assisted suicide and medical killing, or euthanasia, more and more available and accepted. In this country, assurances will be given that the proposed safeguards are firm and reliable. Rarely has this been the case. This proposed change in the law may be a source of relief to some. But it will bring great fear and trepidation to many, especially those who have vulnerabilities and those living with disabilities. What is now proposed will not be the end of the story. It is a story better not begun.

The second point is this: a right to die can become a duty to die.

A law which prohibits an action is a clear deterrent. A law which permits an action changes attitudes: that which is permitted is often and easily encouraged. Once assisted suicide is approved by the law, a key protection of human life falls away. Pressure mounts on those who are nearing death, from others or even from themselves, to end their life in order to take away a perceived burden of care from their family, for the avoidance of pain, or for the sake of an inheritance.

I know that, for many people, there is profound fear at the prospect of prolonged suffering and loss of dignity. Yet such suffering itself can be eased. Part of this debate, then, must be the need and duty to enhance palliative care and hospice provision, so that there can genuinely be, for all of us, the prospect of living our last days in the company of loved ones and caring medical professionals. This is truly dying with dignity. Indeed, the radical change in the law now being proposed risks bringing about for all medical professionals a slow change from a duty to care to a duty to kill.

The third point is this: being forgetful of God belittles our humanity.

The questions raised by this bill go to the very heart of how we understand ourselves, our lives, our humanity. For people of faith in God - the vast majority of the population of the world - the first truth is that life, ultimately, is a gift of the Creator. Our life flows from God and will find its fulfilment in God. 'The Lord gave, and the Lord has taken away; blessed be the name of the Lord.' (Job 1:21) To ignore or deny this truth is to separate our humanity from its origins and purpose. We are left, floating free, detached, in a sphere that lacks firm anchors or destiny, thinking that we can create these for ourselves according to the mood of the age, or even of the day.

The clearest expression of this faith is that every human being is made in the image and likeness of God. That is the source of our dignity and it is unique to the human person. The suffering of a human being is not meaningless. It does not destroy that dignity. It is an intrinsic part of our human journey, a journey embraced by the Eternal Word of God, Christ Jesus himself. He brings our humanity to its full glory precisely through the gateway of suffering and death.

We know, only too well, that suffering can bring people to a most dreadful state of mind, even driving them to take their own lives, in circumstances most often when they lack true freedom of mind and will, and so bear no culpability. But this proposed legislation is quite different. It seeks to give a person of sound will and mind the right to act in a way that is clearly contrary to a fundamental truth: our life is not our own possession, to dispose of as we feel fit. This is not a freedom of choice we can take for ourselves without undermining the foundations of trust and shared dignity on which a stable society rests.

As this debate unfolds, then, I ask you to play your part in it. Write to your MP. Have discussions with family, friends and colleagues. And pray. Please remember: be careful what you wish for; the right to die can become a duty to die; being forgetful of God belittles our humanity.

May God bless us all at this critical time

✠ Cardinal Vincent Nichols

Archbishop of Westminster

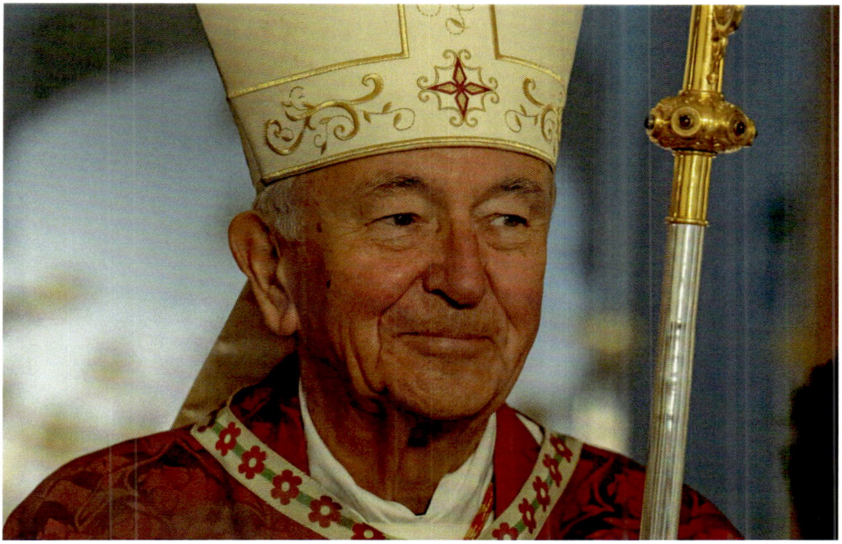

Introduction

When you, your relatives or friends receive an "End of Life" diagnosis, there is a special quality of care offered by a team of specially trained doctors, nurses and support staff including Chaplaincy. What is it called? It is called Hospice Care.

Some of us may be unaware that there are two hundred and twenty hospices providing care in England and Wales for adults. There are also fifty hospices especially for infants and young adults, offering support at what is an important and challenging time.

Many hospices offer day care facilities which you can visit to find out the best care available for a patient, family member or friend. All hospice care is provided for those in need, be they people of faith or none.

In this book, Father Michael Stack shares his relationship as a Hospice Chaplain with many patients who inspired him in his sixteen years in this special ministry. He became aware of the real love and care given by those who minister to people at the end of their life care pathway.

Listening, laughing, crying and touch importantly bring an awareness of intimacy shared by those giving direct care and those receiving hospice care.

This is a journey shared by many who bring support when needed. Yes, it is not a journey of failure but one of true hope.

Acknowledgements

Bernard Longley, Archbishop of Birmingham

Canon Tom Farrell, Parish Priest, Christ the King, Coventry

Madeleine and John Shakespeare

Fiona McLintock, Christ the King Parish Secretary

Dr Patricia O'Brien and family

Father Michael Gamble

Con McHugh

Tom and Mary Manning

Father John Kelly Director of Pastoral Care Tallaght University Hospital Dublin Ireland

Macmillan and Marie Curie Nurses

Hospice Staff and Volunteers

Hospice Chaplains

The Executive Committee of the Association of Catholic Nurses of England and Wales

Catholic Bishops' Conference of England and Wales (Prayer of St Joseph)

Contents

Emma - Respite Care

I'm sat in an armchair watching the colour TV on the wall, and there is Commander Tim Peake in space floating around in zero gravity, after arriving at the International Space Station and with his camera on board he shows us the earth in all its beauty – deep blue and brilliant white clouds. He and his team of astronauts are speeding at 26,000 miles an hour, circling the earth 3000 times, travelling a total of 78 million miles.

At the same time, I'm also watching Emma, a patient in the local hospice. Emma in her 40s. I look around her bed. It's very much like a hospital bed. This is a single room – comfortable with lunch about to arrive. A nurse places a trolley in front of Emma and asks her what she would like to eat, "it's minced meat pie or tomato soup". Emma's favourite is the tomato soup. "Would you like a scoop of ice-cream". Again, Emma goes for the ice-cream. "Any flavour, please".

Emma can see the garden from her bed. There are lots of flowers – lots of colour. Yes, a world of colour.

Emma tells me that she misses the children that she teaches. Fixed to the wall with tape are many 'Get Well' cards. Most have been made individually by pupils at her primary school.

Emma's mother has been looking after her for the last 3 months. The respite care she is receiving in the hospice gives her mum some time to herself and a 10-day break from the daily tasks she has taken on as her carer.

Emma explains to me that she has developed pancreatic cancer. She is on a course of chemotherapy. Lunch arrives. Sister puts the plate onto the tray in from of her, then stares at me! This is the code for me to leave. "Goodbye Emma. I will visit again", "Please do, Father Michael, and thank you for visiting me. Mum will be calling by this afternoon, as will the Head of my school", "Bye, say hello to mum for me"

Emma is eating but the portions are smaller. The care she received is good. Physio calls to make an appointment. Booked for tomorrow.

Next day. Having signed in I knock on Emma's door but no answer. She's with the physio. Sister sees me and invites me to see her privately. This is about a newly arrived patient who may want to see me.

Emma is wheeled back to her room. She's exhausted. As I sit next to Emma, her doctor walks into to room to share some news with her. The only way you would recognise the doctor is by her lanyard, her photo and the stethoscope round her neck. "You can go home on Friday, Emma." We are happy with your condition." Emma was so pleased she burst into tears. Good news is very contagious. I burst into tears, as did the nurse caring for Emma. Tissues all around. The TV is on, and they are showing the Tim Peake story again.

"Father Michael, please give me a blessing before you go." This done, I also prayed for our beautiful world. I prayed for Emma's mum, the support team, all in the hospice and all home carers.

Next stop – Home.

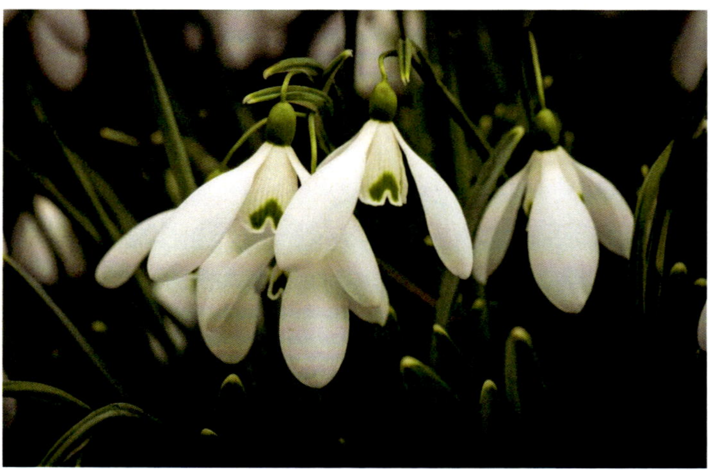

Jim - "I'm a Devout Atheist"

"What do you want?" "Whatever it is, I don't want it, and I'm a devout atheist. Go away." A very pleasing introduction. "Hello, I'm one of the Chaplains. Is that your dog?" "Yes and what has it got to do with you? It's a highland terrier." This dog is curled up at the end of the bed asleep. "I had a friend who had the same breed. She'd fetched it from a kennel – it was four years old. As she introduced the dog to me it decided to bite me on the index finger. There was blood and so a visit to the A & E department for a jab and four stitches" "Don't worry, Patch will not hurt you." I said "He's very passive. How old is Patch?" "Seven years old and he's always with me." I put my hand out to shake hands and said, "From one human being to another, hello." Our hands met and I sat next to Patch stroking him "What is Patch's owners name?" "I'm Jim, what's yours?" "I'm Father Michael." "Do you go round and visit anyone?" "Yes, if folks want to talk. I usually visit at the end of supper time. Have you had some food, Jim?" "Yes, I had some sandwiches – could have taken the crusts off!" "Do you want me to tell the staff nurse?" "Would you?" "Yes. There's ice-cream – jelly – cream cakes and later the drinks trolly if you wish?" "Did you arrive yesterday, Jim?" "Yes, I was transferred from the Walsgrave (UHCW) from the Oncology Ward." "Are any relatives visiting you Jim?" "Yes, tomorrow. My sister and her two children. Do I look a sight, Father Michael? I think the children will be scared as they have never been in a hospice before." "Don't worry Jim, the staff will help reassure them. Tell the staff nurse, that's the one in the light blue uniform after lunch and she will show your family around" "Well, thanks for that Will you visit Patch and me again?"

I told Jim I was around most days. "Let the Staff Nurse know that you want a visit and I will see you on my next visit" "Some folks do see you as a threat, especially if you have a clerical collar on." Listening is the key to a visit to someone like Jim.

Jim and I became good friends and Patch too. A few chocolate nibbles for Patch helped the friendship. Jim explained to me one night that his father sent him and his brother to a Christian school. This, he said, went against the grain. Both were physically punished as they didn't know the Bible. As Jim told me "They were the least Christian folk he'd ever met and turned me against any form of religious witness. You are different Father Michael – can I call you Michael?" "Yes, please do." I said.

In our conversation Jim told me he had been baptised. He also told me he was forced to be Confirmed at school all against his will. Yes, he was an angry person and this all affected his life.

"Father Michael, can we go to the Chapel?" I was rather shocked. "Of course, yes."

First, I found a wheelchair. Next, I got permission off Staff Nurse to relocate. This done, one of the nurses helped move Jim from the bed to the wheelchair. Once done, I wheeled Jim, with Patch sat on his lap, into the Chapel. Jim said straight away how quiet and peaceful the place was. I placed Jim near the Altar overlooking a coloured window. Patch decided to sniff out this place that he had not been in before.

I sat behind Jim having assured him I was present. "What is the window about?" he asked. "The figure is Mary, Jesus' Mother, Jim." "I never knew my mother, Father Michael. I was adopted at 9 years old. I've missed out on life. I don't know who my blood mother was." "Jim, has that been with you all through your life?" "Yes, I have always felt incomplete – and in many ways unloved. To be given away as if I was a chattel." "Tell me Jim, what did you do work wise? Did you use your gifts to help others?" "Yes, I was a male nurse and worked in Liverpool for many years. I saw the suffering many go through and rejected anyone who had a clerical collar or who worked in Chaplaincy. You appear to be different." "How?" "Well, you want to listen to me, and you haven't challenged me as soon as I said I am an atheist!" "Jim, your story of your life is important – that's why I want to listen to you." "Tell me, Father Michael, why do you and your type pray?" "Well, Jim, prayer is like asking and wanting to place issues with the Lord and bringing these to Mary. the Mother of Mothers - Jesus' Mother". "I like the face of Mary in the stain glass window. She looks approachable." "Jim, tell me what you would wish in prayer?" "I wish that I can have a peaceful death here. I have suffered much in my life; all I want is to thank the Macmillan Nurses and all who are here in the hospice for their Care." "Jim, may your prayers be answered – that is what I pray for you- if you are happy to allow me to say this to you?" "You may, but what will happen to Patch? Who will look after him?" "Don't worry about that. I realised that Jim and I had covered much in our chats. In some ways it was Jim who trusted me, a Chaplain, the very type he had a dislike for.

As time went on our friendship developed. I asked Jim if I could give him a blessing. This was new to him – even praying the Lord's Prayer gave him a sense of purpose. Although he did ask me where I got these words from.

Jim's life ended at 2.30pm on Tuesday. He'd had a sandwich to eat. By chance, I called in to see him. As I shook his hand to reach him in his bed, he fell back into silence. I called the nurse, Ella, who tidied the bed. Patch started pining, knowing his master had died.

I gave a final blessing to Jim who was now at peace. Many steps had been made by Jim and all who knew him. May he Rest in Peace.

(Patch was adopted by Ella – Jim's nurse)

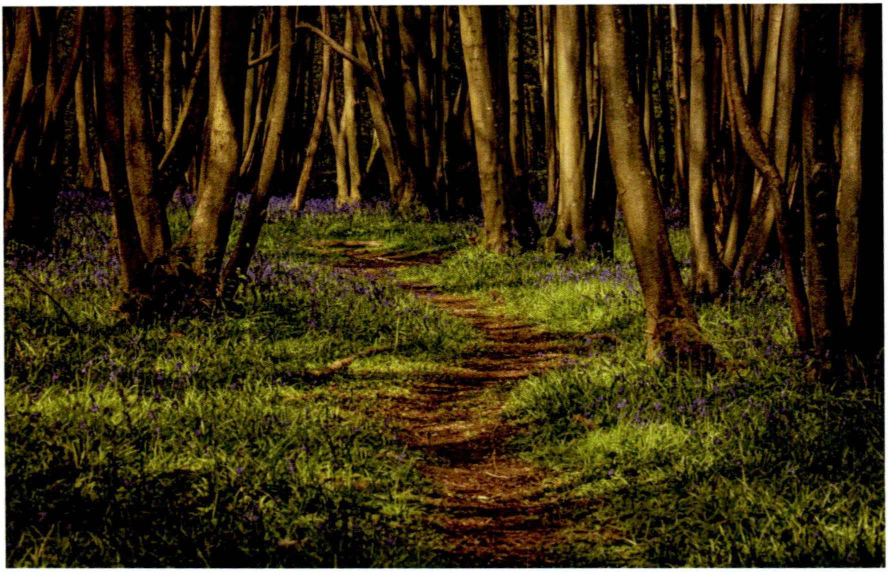

Amanda - Life Saving Dialysis

Dialysis was her life saver. Treatment started a week after Amanda arrived at the Dialysis Unit at the NHS City Hospital where she spent 4 hours having her blood purified. Everything circled around staying alive. Now she could not go on holiday. She had to give up her teaching post.

Amanda's focus was ensuring she arrived on time for her slot. There were 160 beds in the Dialysis Unit. For six days a week these machines and the staff kept everyone alive.

Sunday was the day of rest for the Dialysis machine and for the staff. Not for the maintenance staff, who were also life savers, as they worked on a Sunday to prepare the machines for the Monday morning start again.

As a renal patient, a fistula or graft is taped into place, usually on the hand. After the dialysis, the needle is removed, and a plaster is applied to prevent bleeding. Once over, Amanda can usually go home. Side effects are feeling sick and dizzy. You may have muscle cramps during the procedure.

Sometimes as a short-term measure, or in an emergency, you may be given a neck line, where a small tube is inserted into a vein in your neck.

As well as her family, her faith was important to Amanda. During dialysis I would bring Holy Communion to her. With the curtain pulled around the bed, there was time to pray together. You can be close as you pray together.

Over time, dialysis takes its toll on the patient. Yes, the purifying of blood has a cost. At some point the veins begin to weaken and collapse and the lifesaving event 3 times a week becomes less effective.

Having known Amanda for six years, I was aware the treatment would eventually stop. She shared with me what she wanted to do. She told me that she had visited the Hospice Day Care facilities. Amanda saw the facilities and met some of the staff at the Hospice. Her impressions were that staff were both supportive and caring. This is what she wanted.

Maybe you have never visited a hospice? Most hospices have a Day Care Unit. You can visit – talk to the staff, have lunch. This can help understand the care offered by a local hospice.

It was the second day that Amanda asked to see me. As I arrived into her room her doctor said hello to me as she was leaving. The lanyard ID around her neck and the stethoscope was her identity. "Can I have a chat with you, Father Michael when you leave?" Amanda was very calm. Her sister had visited her and she seemed content. She had eaten a few fries and mushy peas. The remains were on the plate.

"Any pain, Amanda?" "No Father" she answered. "Have you got a sweet tooth?" "Sometimes, yes." Having left Amanda, I called into the main office where Doctor Sue wanted a chat. I sat down and Sue briefed me. "I think Amanda is comfortable. She's in no pain. I think she will be with us for maybe two weeks." "OK" I said, "will her system close down?" "She will stop eating then she will slowly experience pain issues, which we can help with. We will talk to her sister and let her know. Amanda is fully aware as I have discussed this with her." "Thank you doctor." What next? Amanda wanted me to pray with her. As I sat with her, I asked in prayer for the Lord to be with her. "Lord, help her to be strong, and help those who are caring for her."

The doctors estimate of two weeks, turned out to be three days. Amanda had watched an episode of Eastenders and said she was in pain. The caring staff were aware she was on the final cycle and asked her if she wanted family to be called. All she asked was that I was called.

Upon arrival, I could see Amanda was semi-conscious. I gave her the Sacrament of the Sick – that is the laying on of hands on her head and anointing with oil the Sign of the Cross on her forehead and the palms of her hands. As I prayed the Lord's Prayer, she turned her head and died.

Staff Nurse immediately burst into tears and called for assistance. There was nothing else we could do. Staff Nurse phoned the family, and they arrived 5 minutes later. I waited to see them. I offered my condolences, said a prayer and left them. I returned to the main hospital, and the Sister on the Renal Unit asked what had just happened. She said she would let the staff who cared for her know.

I became aware that Amanda was at rest. The family later informed me they were grateful that I was present at her death.

Can we and do we prepare for our last hours? Some, yes – some, no! All I know is, Amanda's struggles are over. She received tender loving care, right up to the end of her life.

May she Rest in Peace.

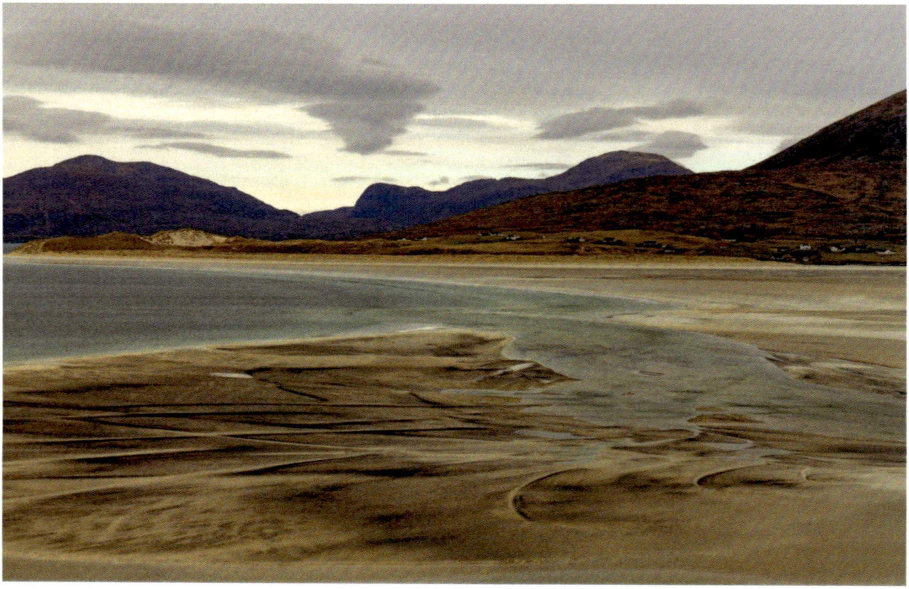

Michael - at Peace

Just as I walked into the front door of the Hospice, paramedics were bringing Michael in on a stretcher, with his partner and most of his belongings from the ward, in what's known as a transfer.

The patient was calmly taken to what appeared to be a comfortable room, with everything that could be needed, even a colour TV.

For some, the word "hospice" instils fear. For Michael, he was full of relief. Why? As he had waited for three days for this transfer.

His carers introduced themselves, so did I briefly. It was just a quick hello.

Like all patients, Michael's notes were looked at by a doctor, who would brief the staff on what medication the patient was receiving.

Michael was comfortable. His appetite was also good. His family and friends were able to visit at any time day or night.

During the day a doctor would visit him and review his needs with the nursing staff.

When we met, Michael asked me "Do you visit regularly, Father?" "I'm here at any time that suits you. Maybe you want a chat? Maybe you want a prayer, or the sacraments? Just ask."

Pain control had become an issue. Now Michael was reassured that his pain could be resolved.

On one visit, supper was about to be served. One of the nurses invited Michael to have a sherry before his meal. He said yes and the drink was duly prepared in from of him. Sherry stimulates the taste buds and helps the appetite.

Sometimes, Michael found this amusing. I arrived just before supper, to which I was asked if I would have sherry too. "Many thanks, but I'm not allowed – on duty and all that!"

With regular visiting you get to know each other. So any worries do come to the surface.

On one visit, Michael told me that he had not been a good father to some of his children. I listened carefully, being non-judgemental. One of his sons refused to visit him in hospital. This concerned him greatly. "Father Michael, am I a failure?" to which I responded, "You have done your best, bringing up three children is not easy, you have worked many years to support your family. If you didn't love them, you would not have done this." This reply seemed to help Michael, who asked me for a blessing. "I'm not religious, Father Michael, but I need some help here." "I am here, and I will help" I said.

Another four visits gave Michael a deep sense of calm and acceptance.

I was called in to visit him at 4.00am. The family were present. As I arrived into the room, the family were round the bedside. Michael was not responding. His daughter was holding his hand. I quietly said the Lord's Prayer. Everyone joined in and Michael died peacefully. It was like he was asleep. Yes, there were tears. I withdrew, as did the nurse looking after him.

We had a conversation about Michael. The nurse caring for him shed a few tears. Nurse Jean knew about the difficultly with Michael's children. Although his son refused to visit his father in hospital, he did visit him in the hospice.

After an hour, I returned to the room. The eldest daughter grabbed my hand and thanked me as she shook my hand, "You have given dad an inner peace that he didn't have before. On behalf of the family, we thank you, and the staff here."

May he Rest in Peace.

Lord, thank you for the nurses who care for patients like Michael. May all who minister to the sick in our hospices be supported when life draws to a close. May family and friends also be aware they too are not alone as they grieve for their loved ones. Amen.

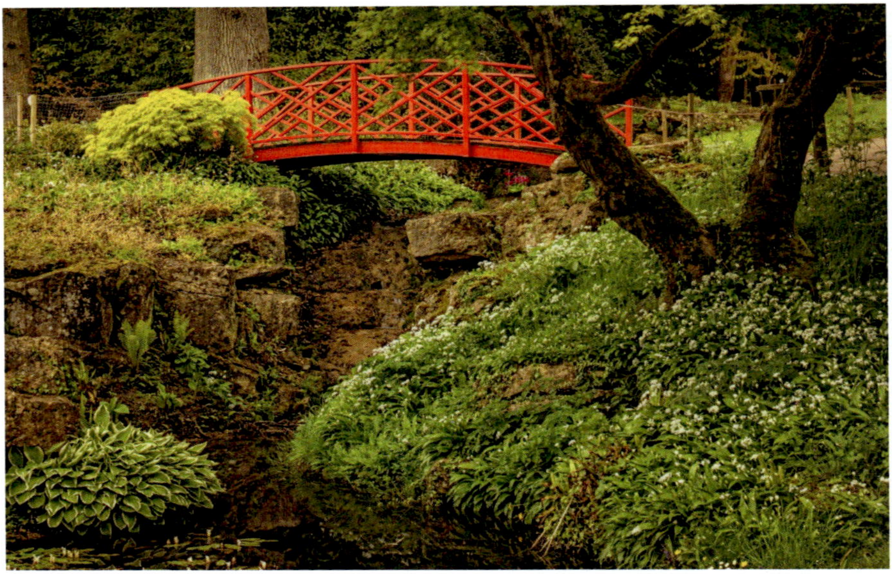

Toni - Forgiveness

"Look here, Father Michael, since we last spoke, I've heard nothing from the family that I am estranged from. What have you done or heard?"

I told Toni that I had made contact with her sister and explained to her that Toni was receiving hospice care. I let her know that she could visit at any time, day or night. I contacted Toni's mother, Janice, and explained that time was short, and she could visit at any time. Both relatives lived locally. That was not the problem. There was hurt on both sides. Things had been expressed and forgiveness was not on the table, as they say.

How does one try to bring warring families together when damage has caused such pain?

Toni was listening to some music on her mobile "What are you listening to?" I asked. "It's Ed Sheeran, Father Michael." "Oh yes, who's he?" "Blimey, Father Michael, you're so out of date!"

"Toni, tell me how are you? Put the mobile phone down, and let me switch the TV off too." Now there was quiet. Toni could think about what was important. "I want my family, Father Michael". Tears ran down Toni's face. I picked up a tissue and offered it to her. There was a knock on the door. I said, "Come in, please." It was Toni's mother, Janice. As soon as she saw Toni in tears, she instantly burst into tears herself. "I will leave you" I said "Please talk." I withdrew, closing the door quietly. What followed was a daughter and her mother hugging each other with many, many more tears.

Leaving them an hour, I slowly returned with two cups of tea. Mum, Janice and Toni were talking, looking at a picture of Toni that her mum had brought to show Toni. Yes, there was guilt on both sides. Toni said, "Father Michael, we have seen faults on both sides, we had tried not to back down, as it was the other's fault. Who taught you how to make a good cup of tea?" I found the atmosphere clearing in the room. Janice was fully aware that Toni is not going to improve. Toni had shown the syringe driver to her mum. She didn't quite understand what this was for.

Supper was about to be served. Mum was now settled and stayed with Toni overnight She decided to sleep in the armchair. Supper was offered to her, fish fingers and mashed potatoes, followed by ice cream. I didn't stay.

The following day Toni asked to see me and asked me to take her and her Mum to the chapel. It was quiet. There Toni and Janice sat and were able to think about the past. Where had the time gone - where had the years gone? All those lost birthdays – those lost Christmases – those lost anniversaries. "Have you a prayer book, Father Michael?" "Use this, Toni, it's my anointing book, it has a list of saints whom you can pray to and ask them for help. There is a section (Litany) of forgiveness. We all need to be forgiven and to forgive, don't we?"

As the silence in the chapel was broken by the arrival of a patient in a wheelchair being pushed by her carer, by instinct we all stared at them. Once settled, our attention returned to Toni and her mother. Toni began to tell me about of her complicated journey through life. Toni then turned to me, and asked if my journey was like hers?" I said "Yes and no" "What does that mean?" I briefly explained that I joined the St Vincent de Paul Society, and became the local president. I was only 23 years old. Their role was to pray together and visit the sick and the poor in a parish. I told Toni, I became aware of the iniquity in our society. I told Toni I was working for a millionaire who only cared about money. I thought there was more to life than helping make money for someone who already had too much, but little care for others. My journey in the priesthood was not easy – "nothing" is easy in life, Toni – Don't we all know this?

I forced the conversation back to Toni. She was more composed and responsive with her mother.

Suddenly, the syringe driver began to bleep. This meant that the morphine container was empty. We returned to Toni's room – mum pushing Toni in her wheelchair.

Alas, my memory of Toni blurs as she was one of many, who asked for someone representing the church to listen to her fractured and bruised life. I remained with Toni, praying together. Her mum joined. She died peacefully in the hospice. Her local priest held a brief service at the local crematorium. Her nurse, who shared much time with Toni in the hospice, was present, and the family said their farewell.

May she Rest in Peace.

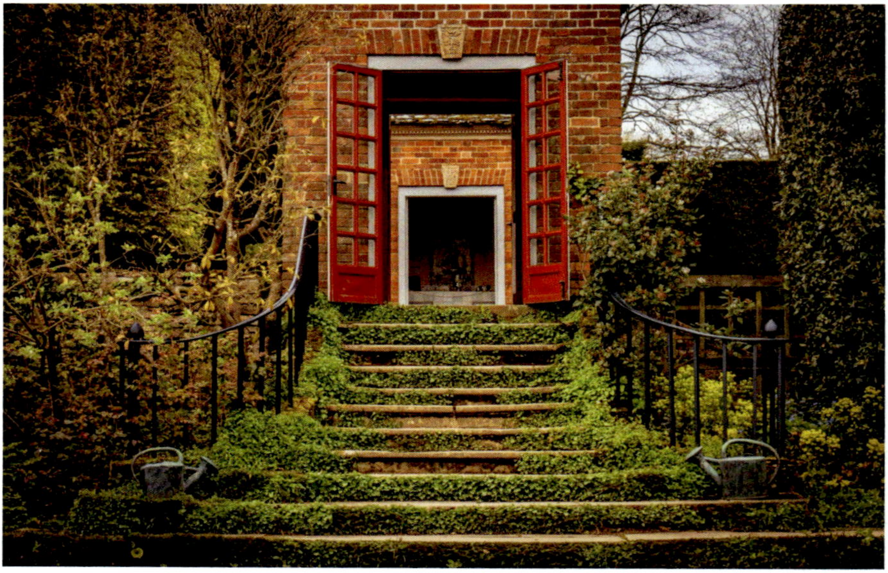

Peter - Cancer leads to conversion

Peter was 75 years of age, but didn't lock it. Born in the Rhondda Valley in Wales, Peter left school and joined the Royal Air Force as a Rear Gunner in Bomber Command. After the Second World War, Peter met Molly and married her. They settled down and had a family (three children).

I met Peter on ward North 3A in the city hospital. This was the oncology ward. Peter had a cancerous tumour in the brain. I had just visited a young man who had been receiving chemotherapy for testicular cancer that can be treated, if detected earlier. Peter waved me over to his bedside. He sat in a chair with his day clothes on, and on his head, he wore a cloth cap.

Upon asking Peter how he was, he immediately asked me if I was a Catholic Priest. As I said yes to his question, he began to tell me his story. During World War II he had met the Catholic RAF Padre. He was very much encouraged by him. Peter told me he was on the bombing raid of Hiroshima, Japan. He told me that Leonard Cheshire was his Squadron Leader. This was when the first Nuclear Bomb was dropped, killing 140,000 people. For many years these actions, as well as Cologne and Hamburg played on his mind. There was much guilt. I tried to explain to him that decisions and orders were given and carried out in times of war. Yes, his actions had caused deaths but had also saved many lives.

Peter blamed himself for these actions and burst into tears. He was still deeply affected by this series of events from many years ago. Staff nurse arrived at the bedside to give Peter a new unit of chemotherapy. She disconnected the line from Peter's neck vein and put a new bag of what seemed like a clear bag of gin fluid, onto a steel pole with four wheels on it. Peter could move about for a while - but once reconnected he would grip the steel pole and wheel it around with him. Peter was fully aware that he was dying.

Three days later I met Peter again. This time Molly, his wife, was present. Peter was in the chair and Molly was sat on the bed. I shook hands with both of them and edged my way towards the bed. As I sat on the bed Molly immediately led the conversation. She told me that Peter wanted to be received into the Catholic Church. But what kind of process was involved? I told Peter and Molly that a short period of instruction would follow and then reception into the church. Molly was trying to get a time programme from me. It was arranged to have short twenty-minute chats with Peter when he felt able. After a prayer and a blessing for both, I went to speak to the Sister in charge about Peter's progress. Sister was sitting in the office studying a patient's file chart. Sister Jane looked up as I asked about Peter's prognosis.

'About three months' was the answer. There wasn't much time. 'Would Peter be staying on the ward till the end?' I asked. 'No, he will be transferred to a hospice in two weeks', said Sister. 'Does his wife know?' 'Yes' replied Jane. I thanked her for the information.

What followed was a period of Catechesis over six weeks. Molly was present and as Peter listened to me, she too showed great attention. With the move to the Hospice my task became easier. Mainly because there were no interruptions, and we had a quiet room too. Lots of cups of tea and biscuits were also greatly received.

It was during the instruction that Peter told me he had wanted to become Catholic for many years, and that I was the instrument to help him. I felt very humble. Very ill patients have a habit of wanting something familiar to them to touch. One of Peter's neighbours was a patient at the hospice and had his little Jack Russel dog on his bed each night. Some would want a soft toy, a neck chain, a picture or even a blanket from home. With Peter it was his flat cap. It was on his head all the time, day or night.

When it came to the reception of Peter into the Church, we used the hospice lounge. Peter recited the Apostles Creed. I then Confirmed him, anointed him and gave him Holy Communion. None of the family present or staff were Catholics, but they said afterwards how profoundly moving the ceremony had been for them. Yes that cloth cap was removed by Molly, for the laying on of hands, and then put back on.

Peter died peacefully two weeks later. Molly told me that something had changed in Peter after the reception ceremony. She said that he had received an inner peace, which she could visibly see in him. Molly expressed her thanks for the prayers we would say together in the hospital and in the hospice. She asked me what the prayer was, that we kept had saying as I prayed over Peter. It was the Lord's Prayer.

After a brief Church service in Birmingham, we took Peter's body back home to the Rhondda Valley. Our journey took three hours. The family carried the coffin up a steep hill overlooking a once scarred valley, now returned to its rich green. Peter's remains were put to rest next to his parents. This was his wish too. May he Rest in Peace. Amen.

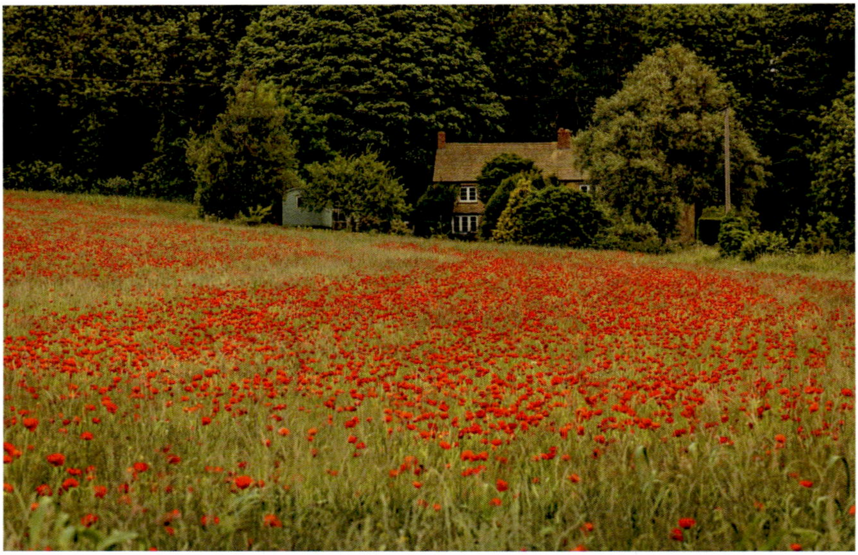

Tommy – Mum, Dad and Teddy!

It was a call to visit Tommy who was five years of age.

I first met him in the company of his parents in the hospice.

They explained to me that Tommy had received six sessions of treatment (radiation therapy). Looking at him, he was bubbly, blue eyed and fidgeting on mum's lap. Now he was staring at me. He looked like any ordinary child, except for the tube into his nose telling me he had a serious condition. Tommy had in his hands his teddy, who remained with him, always. Teddy was a bit worn. His paws and face were threadbare. Tommy offered him to me. Mum said "Father Michael, will you give Teddy a blessing?" My response was "of course – we bless Teddy and all his friends – all those who live with Teddy."

I know where mum was heading as she said, "Can Tommy have a blessing too?" "Yes, of course." I asked if I could put my hand on Tommy's head, just like I did with Teddy. "Please do" said Dad. As I put my hand above Tommy's head, he was quite afraid of this action. But soon fear changed to acceptance as he shouted out for Teddy to be with him. Yes, the worn Teddy's face and paws had been hugged with much love. Teddy, like his Mum and Dad were close and the love they showed for Tommy was real. The burdens of illness in Tommy reflected in his parents, who were now aware that the hospice care would come to a conclusion, losing the one they loved – Tommy. Nursing care was exemplary. Tommy would go into the playroom, where other children played with the many toys, all donated to the children's hospice. Doctor Jan briefed me and explained there would be no further treatment. As Tommy deteriorated both parents moved in, sleeping facilities were always available and they were supported by the caring hospice staff.

This was one of the 50 hospices in England for children and young adults, all available to support those in need of support and care with life limiting or life-threatening conditions, and their families. Included in all of this is support for parents and siblings.

It was at 9pm on a Friday that Tommy suddenly held Mum and Dad's hands and then he died. Yes, Teddy was also present. I prayed for Tommy with his parents. The nurse looking after Tommy left in tears. Now Tommy was at rest. A very young life had ended.

Two weeks later, Tommy's parents' parish priest (Father Patrick) held a service in their local church. Also present was Teddy – flowers – cards – balloons and two hundred folks from the community, all supporting and saying farewell to a loved child. Father Patrick's scripture reading was "Think of the love the Father has lavished on us by letting us be called God's children, for that is what we are."

Tommy's bravery lives on through his parents love for him. May he Rest in Peace.

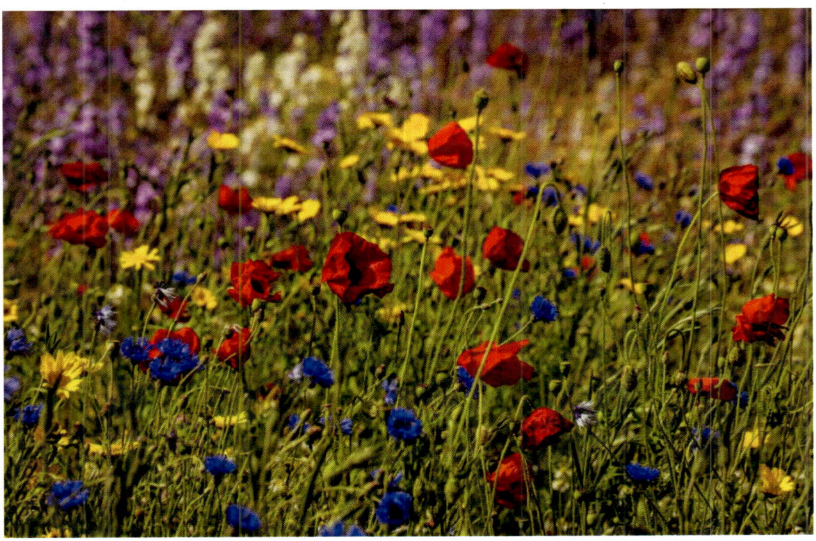

Rav - HIV Aids

At the age of 26 Rav had much to reflect on. His parents had rejected him when he was sixteen. It was because he not only handled drugs but also took them. From the age of fourteen Rav frequently came into contact with the police, and he had spent three years in jail for selling hard drugs.

I first met Rav in the Hospice. He had his own room and was very open to any visits. At the nursing station I found out why Rav was in Hospital. Sister gently lowered her voice and said that Rav was a HIV Aids patient. She asked me, would I be visiting him after giving me this information. I informed Sister I had just visited him, and would see him again. Rav's background was Pakistani by birth, and Muslim by faith.

When either the drugs trolley, or lunch was brought to Rav, he would respond to the interaction. A visit meant a lot to him. I remember listening to Rav about his prison experiences. He recalled to me that he asked to see a Catholic priest, when in Winson Green Prison. When I asked why he made such a request, he told me it was because previously a Catholic priest had listened to him. The priest has listened to his story and had not judged him.

Rav's childhood had been a very unhappy one. Physical violence and sexual abuse had left its mark on him. The escape to the drug culture subsequently led him to prison life. Every time I visited, Rav would ask for a prayer. I would pray over him and then place my hand upon his head and bless him. Rav would frequently cry. To which I would ask, what was the matter? Simply, Rav had not felt the touch of another upon him, by someone who was non-threatening.

Rav felt that his life had been a failure. He said he caused so much pain and worry to his parents. He felt that there was no way that he could make up for this, or that his parents could ever forgive him. Deep down he wanted to be forgiven. But how? In the conversation that followed I suggested that Rav write down on paper what he wanted forgiveness for, and by whom. He became agitated by this request. As I built up a relationship with Rav, I asked him to give me the piece of paper with his details on. He asked me what I would do with it. I explained simply that I would not read it but place it in a special place in the Church and pray for all those Rav felt he had most hurt, asking for forgiveness. I also said that Rav's creator would see his heart, accept his genuine forgiveness, and offer pardon to him.

Rav held my hand as I sat by the bedside and told me that if this could be accomplished, he would feel so different about his past. We parted with a prayer and a blessing. I asked the Lord in my prayer to restore the hearts of those whose past had been so damaged, asking also for forgiveness for all involved, Rav again wept as I left. This time as I left something struck me. He was a different person from the man I met just six weeks ago. Two days later I called again to see Rav. His bed was empty. I called at the nurse's station and casually asked where Rav had been moved to. Did I not know that Rav died, last night at about 1am? Two of the nurses were with him. They had just changed his sheets, and he had asked them to hold his hands as he died peacefully.

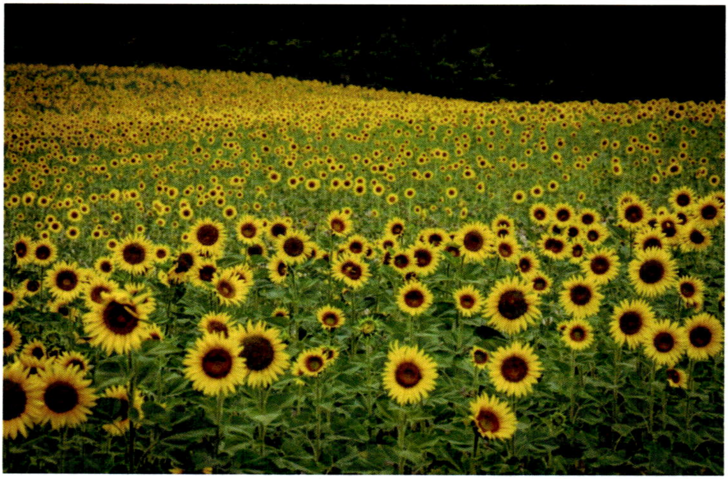

Sarah - Marriage by Emergency

Every so often you meet a patient who is bubbly and out-going in nature. Sarah was such a case. Although only 32 years of age, she knew that little could be done to stop cancer in her stomach. The ten sessions of chemotherapy were over. The only possible next step was to try and insert a tube, which could give a few more months to her short life.

I met Sarah while she was receiving treatment on the oncology ward. As warned beforehand, her blond hair fell out after session two. She now wore a scarf to hide her baldness. She once told me when the scarf was off that she thought she looked like Sinead O'Connor. Regularly, Sarah would give me the signal that she was about to vomit. I would inform Staff Nurse, who would attend to her. Sarah informed me, whilst visiting the ward, that her doctor had advised her to be transferred to the Hospice. This was so that they could control her pain. Sarah agreed and so the task of moving this frail young woman began. The hospice was only two miles from the hospital. So, Sarah was carefully carried into an ambulance. With a police escort (two motor bikes), the journey took 25 minutes as the ambulance travelled at ten miles as hour. Awaiting at the hospice was a special air bed so she would be bed sore free.

Now Sarah was receiving morphine intravenously, by a syringe driver. This small machine pumps morphine into the veins to stop pain. On day five at the hospice, Sarah was cheerful but becoming weak. Her weight loss was now of concern to all. It was suggested that an x-ray be carried out to see if that tube could be inserted. If so, maybe three months life could help Sarah. After notifying the police (motorbike escort) an ambulance was booked to take Sarah to City Hospital. This time Sarah's mum was travelling with her. Her mum was a Catholic. She held in her hand a small blue statuette of Mary containing water from the shrine in Lourdes, France. Placed very carefully into the back of the ambulance, Mum clambered up the steps inside the vehicle. The journey took 30 minutes. Upon arrival, Sarah was taken into X-ray where the department was ready. The necessary photos were taken and within half an hour the doctor was able to make a judgement. This procedure could not be done, was the answer. Not to lose this opportunity, Sarah asked the driver of the ambulance for a favour. She wanted him to drive her and her mum to McDonald's. As Sarah was on fluids only, solids were out. Would they allow her this chance? The driver walked towards the police officers and asked them. The answer was yes. But what was it that she wanted? 'Only two strawberry and banana milkshakes', replied Sarah. So picture if you can, an ambulance with its blue flashing lights and two police motorbikes and lights crawling along the Bristol Road at five miles an hour, at midday. The salesman at the drive-thru stared in disbelief at all the blue flashing lights and demanded to be told just what was going on. Four milkshakes were quickly supplied as a gift by McDonald's. The convoy returned back up the Bristol Road, with Sarah a very happy person. Although she had now lost three possible months, she had gained her favourite meal. Sarah had weeks to live. The following day as I sat by her bed, Trevor walked into the room and sat next to me. Trevor was Sarah's boyfriend. Sarah looked at Trevor who jumped up and kissed her. Then he sat down again. Sarah told me that she had a big favour to ask. I assumed that it was another purchase of milkshakes. It was not, this time spiritual help that she required. I anointed Sarah. We said the Lord's Prayer together and she became quite composed. She thanked me for the anointing. She said there was one last request. What was it? 'Will you marry me?'

Within 24 hours the register was contacted and booked. Forms were completed. Trevor, Sarah's partner was ready to be wed. At 11am on Saturday, the guests (approximately 25) assembled in the lounge area. The wedding cake arrived. All was now ready. Sarah was dressed in a flowing gown. As she could no longer walk, she was wheeled into the lounge in a large fold back armchair. This was a special moment for Sarah and Trevor. The ceremony was emotionally charged with everyone willing on Sarah. As five of the staff who were nursing Sarah were present, they too were on edge. No one could remember the last hospice wedding. Both bride and groom answered their promises without mistakes. But when I asked Sarah to honour Trevor ... IN SICKNESS AND IN HEALTH, TILL DEATH DO US PART She looked up at me and said, 'I will think about it.' At this, everyone present just burst into tears. The emotions could no longer be contained. Both the witnesses wept, and all were searching for handkerchiefs - except Sarah and Trevor. They just smiled at each other. Through my tears I asked Sarah to simply say "I do". Which she did. Even the registrar, as the books were being signed, kept wiping his eyes. All hearts were heavy with joy and sadness. Sarah's mum was sobbing uncontrollably. I gently picked up the bouquet of flowers, and threw them towards mum. She quickly caught them, and everyone focussed upon this incident. As the cork popped and the cake was cut, the seriousness of the event faded. Everyone enjoyed Sarah and Trevor's special day - Marriage by Emergency.

On Monday, the wedding photos arrived, and all the staff wanted to browse through them. The wedding was the main topic that week for staff and patients. I agreed that the photos were beautiful. I searched for the one taken as I threw Sarah's bouquet. There it was. After that incident the tension had gone. Thank goodness.

Trevor now spent all his time with his wife. He gave up running his café in the city centre. He loved her and wanted to be with her, now that he knew time was short. On a visit I made, Sarah asked me what she should do with the statuette with water in it. I told her to drink the contents and say a prayer. This she did. After this, she was never sick again.

As the days drew on, Sarah's weight loss increased, and she stopped consuming anything. She became agitated and confused. I called to visit at midnight. Her breathing became shallow. Mum and Trevor were present. Again, I anointed Sarah. Sister began to tidy the sheets and whispered to me 'I think she is going.' As we prayed the Lord's Prayer together, I concluded with the Litany of Saints. As I said, 'St Bernadette of Lourdes, Pray for her', her head slightly turned to the left and her life quietly and calmly ended.

Trevor held her hand and tears dropped onto the sheets and onto her hand. Sister and I withdrew to leave the family with Sarah. All the night staff who had nursed Sarah and cared for her, asked if they could visit and say their goodbyes. Trevor was please for them to do this. Now she was released from the suffering she had endured. For Sarah, her young life was not ended but simply changed.

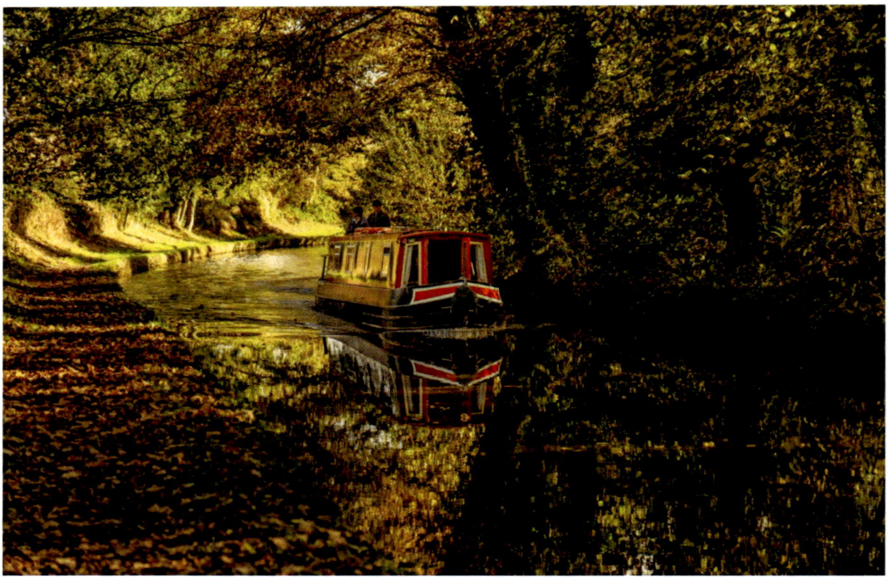

Monica and Marie

As they were soon to retire as nursing sisters, Monica and Marie saw an important need for those who were dying. Special Care should be available for the most vulnerable and those in need of "End of Life Care."

After a meeting with the Archbishop, a place was found, which could be used to become a Hospice in Birmingham. Starting with four beds, Monica and Marie were the starting point to care for those most in need. 1979 began St Mary's Hospice journey for those of faith and no faith. It was with thanks to Monica and Marie's vision to provide the very best care for patients living with life limiting illnesses, and their families and friends.

We sincerely thank Matrons2 Monica Pierce and Marie Hession, for their vision, which became St Mary's Hospice in Birmingham. For the many doctors, nurses, staff, support workers have given their gifts of care to those who lived and died at End of Life – thank you. For the many supporters of the Hospice who gave material help to run the Hospice – thank you. For the many volunteers who gave their time and energy in supporting the running of the Hospice – thank you.

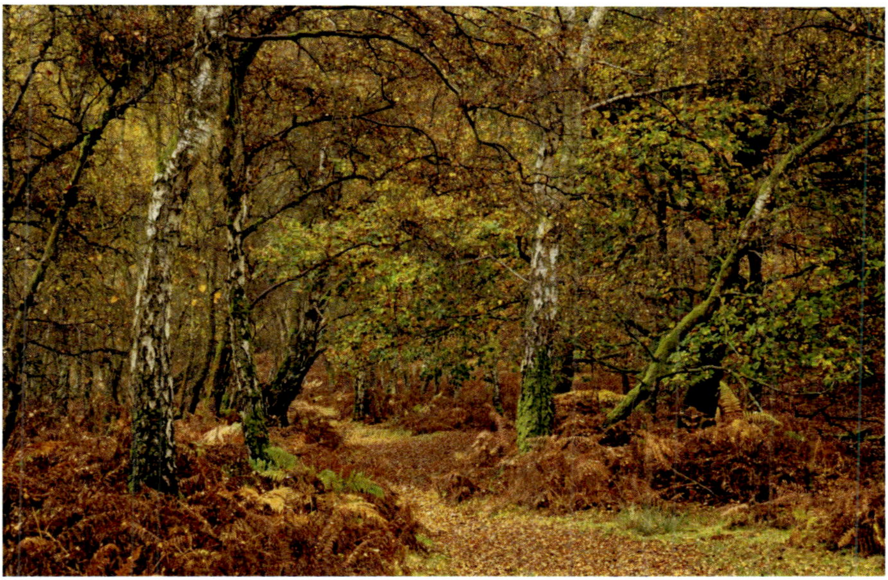

Tributes

Florence Nightingale

Many of us will not be aware that May 12th is the birthday of a woman given the title "The Lady with the Lamp". Born in 1829 in Florence, Italy, of well-to-do parents, Florence became a nurse and went with 38 colleagues to Crimea to care for wounded soldiers. She understood how important it was to keep medical equipment and hospital beds clean to stop disease spreading. She changed the way injured and sick people were treated.

Florence started the first nurse training school in the world.

She stopped the filthy conditions causing diseases and infections – she told all to wash with their hands in hospitals. She introduced cleanliness and compassion.

In 1860 Florence set up a training school at St Thomas' Hospital, London. She wrote a famous book – Notes on Nursing, used to train nurses.

Having heard so much about her, Queen Victoria invited her to Balmoral.

Florence was the first person to produce statistics, with her use of Rose charts – remember this was in the 1850s!

In 1844 she claimed at 16 her wish to minister to the sick was a call from God.

As a pioneer of statistics, she wrote 150 texts. As the founder of modern nursing, she died aged 90, in 1910 as a national hero. She is buried in the village cemetery of St Margaret's Church, East Wellow, in Hampshire. A Memorial Service was held at St Paul's Cathedral, London.

Edith Cavell

Edith was born on 4th December 1865. Her schooling was at home by her parents until she was 16 years of age. Her home was Swardeston, near Norwich where she would deliver food to villagers in need. She was determined through her Christian upbringing to make a difference.

Edith wrote, "Someday, somehow, I am going to do something useful. I don't know what it will be. I only know that it will be something for people."

Edith trained to become a Nurse from 1886 – 1899 at the Royal London Hospital, in East London in 1907 she became a Founding Director of Belgium's first Professional Nurse Training School in Brussels.

In 1914, the Great War began, and Germany invaded Belgium. Edith and her team cared for casualties regardless of their origin or on which side of the war they were fighting. She said any wounded soldier must be treated, friend or foe, each man a father or son. The profession of nurses knows no frontiers.

Edith helped those trained behind enemy lines to escape from Belgium. It was a spy network over 200 allied soldiers escaped. Edith and her team were caught, arrested and imprisoned. After a few days in solitary confinement, Edith was tried and found guilty of treason.

On the afternoon of 11th October 1915, Edith learned that she and four others would be executed by firing squad the next morning. As a Christian, Nurse Edith faced her death with calm courage. She is reported to have said, "I have no fear or shrinking. I have seen death so often it is not strange or fearful for me". That night Edith prayed for forgiveness of those who would kill her. She had no hatred or bitterness towards anyone.

Edith was a beacon of light in a world of war and violence and a true guardian of mercy to all.

She was executed by firing squad on 12th October 1915.

She was buried at Norwich Cathedral in May 1919 after a state funeral at Westminster Abbey.

Cicely Saunders – Founder of Modern Hospice

Cicely was born on 22nd June 1918. She was the eldest with two siblings. Wanting to become a nurse she trained at Nightingale School of Nursing at St Thomas' Hospital in London. She next trained to be a doctor at St Thomas' Medical School (now merged with King's College School of Medical Education).

Cicely said it was whilst nursing at St Joseph's Hospice, a Catholic establishment in Hackney, East London, she researched pain control.

1967 was the beginning of Cicely's first purpose-built hospice. This Hospice was founded on the principles of combining teaching and clinical research, with pain and symptom relief with holistic care to the physical, social, psychological and spiritual needs of its patients and their family and friends.

Cicely's care philosophy was "You matter because you are you, you matter to the last moment of your life." St Christopher's was a place whose patients could wear their own clothes, could garden, write, talk, get their hair done.

In 1977, Cicely was awarded an Honorary Lambeth Doctorate by the Archbishop of Canterbury.

In 2000, Cicely became President of the Hospice.

She was made a Fellow of the Royal College of Surgeons, Physicians and of Nurses.

She was made a Dame of the Order of St Gregory the Great (By the Pope).

Cicely died at the age of 87 in 2005 at St Christopher's Hospice.

St Joseph - Aspirations for The Dying

[To be pronounced in the presence of a dying person]

O God, be gracious to me;
O God, have mercy on me;
O God, forgive me my sins!
O God the Father, have mercy on me;
O Jesus, be gracious to me;
O Holy Spirit, strengthen me!
O God the Father, do not reject me;
O Jesus, do not abandon me;
O God the Holy Spirit, do not forsake me!
O my God, into Thy hands I commend my spirit;
O Jesus, Son of David, have mercy on me!
O Jesus, Son of Mary, have mercy on me!
O Jesus, I believe in Thee;
O Jesus I hope in Thee;
O Jesus, I love Thee!
O Jesus, I place all my trust in Thy bitter Passion!
O Jesus, in Thy Sacred Wounds I hide myself!
O Jesus, I enclose myself in Thy Sacred Heart!

Holy Mary, Mother of God, assist me!
Holy Mary, protect me from the evil spirit!
Holy Mary, turn thine eyes of mercy upon me!
O Mary, Mother of mercy, obtain grace for me from thy dear Son!
Come to my aid, O Mary, in this my anguish and need!
O Mary, enclose me in thy virginal Heart!
O Mary, commend me to thy Son, present me to thy Son,
reconcile me with thy Son!

St. Joseph, obtain for me grace and mercy!
St. Joseph, assist me in my struggle against the enemy of my salvation!
St. Joseph, to thee do I entrust my soul: do thou save it for me!
St. Joseph, remember me, and obtain mercy for me!

O Holy Guardian Angel do not abandon me,
But combat for me and preserve me from the evil one!
My dear Patron Saints, pray for me!
Jesus, Jesus, Jesus, into Thy hands I commend my spirit!

Prayer to St Joseph (Patron Saint of the Dying)

Faithful Joseph, with the fulfilment of the Lord's promise,
you peacefully leave this world in Jesus and Mary's hands.
Your faith transforms death into the sowing of life;
thus, God considers you to be a just man.
Your heart overflows in the presence of the Lord.
With your hands outstretched to God, your night is filled with prayers.
Surrounded by the living, you embark upon the great march to the promise Land.
Open our eyes that we may glimpse the road to Life that lies beyond death.
May nothing, not denial, anger, nor depression, separate us from the Love of God.
Strengthen our faith in God who always finds ways of preserving us in his friendship.
Be beside us to hold our hands when we take our first steps toward the Eternal Kingdom.
Amen

Taken from https://www.cbcew.org.uk/prayers-for-the-sick-and-dying

St Joseph – Guardian and Patron of the sick and the dying. Feast Day on 19th March.

Frequently Asked Questions about Hospices

Q How much does Hospice care cost?
A Nothing. It is free to everyone using the service.

Q What is the aim of Hospice care?
A The aim is to improve the lives of patients who have an incurable illness.

Q What is Holistic care?
A It is respecting the wishes of the person who is ill by looking after their medical, emotional, social, practical, psychological and spiritual needs. This includes the patient's family and carers.

Q Can Hospice care be at home?
A Yes, most Hospice care is provided at home. It also can be provided in a care home or as an inpatient in the Hospice. Hospice care is a style of care rather than something that takes place in a specific building.

Q What is a Hospice team?
A There are health care assistants, doctors, nurses, social workers, therapists, counsellors, chaplains and trained volunteers.

Q What does Hospice care cover?
A Managing pain with other symptoms. Looking after you, so that your carers can have a break from caring for a short while. Information about coping financially and bereavement care and Spiritual and psychological care is available.

Q Can I have a look around a Hospice?
A Yes, the staff will show you around the facilities and be happy to answer any questions. If you have a computer, take a virtual tour.

Q You only need Hospice care when you are dying?
A No. The Hospice team might help control symptoms such as pain or breathlessness early on in your illness- meaning you stay at the Hospice for a few days before going home.

Q How does one get referred to a Hospice?
A Your GP will refer you or your loved ones to a Hospice.

Q Where does funding come from to support our Hospices?
A In England, 33% of funding comes from the state. In Wales, 24% of funding comes from the state. All Hospices are registered as a charity. Fundraising is an important part of income. Hospice shops, taking part in sponsored events, auctions, lotteries, events at Easter and Christmas, donations, Legacies in Wills - all support Hospice funding.

Q What if 24-hour care is needed?
A The patient is moved into a medical facility providing care. Loved ones (family/friends) are offered bereavement and support care when a patient has died.

Q Is there support for infants?
A. Yes. Hospice care is available for children up to five years of age.

More information is available online for example https://www.hospiceuk.org/information-and-support

About Father Michael

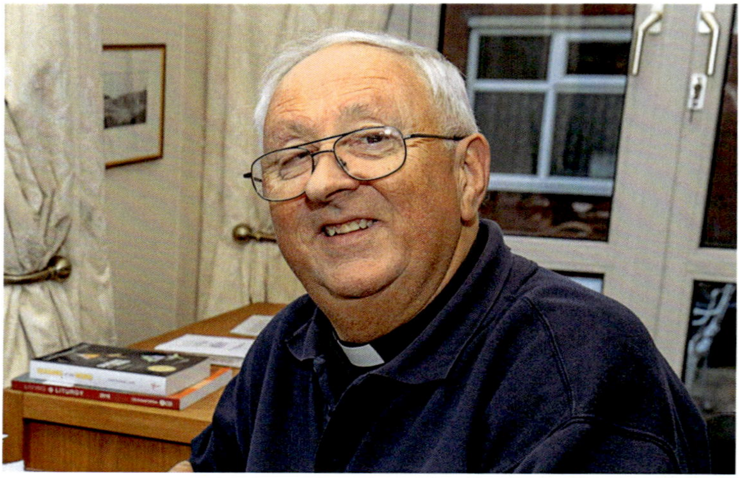

Father Michael Stack was born in Hartlepool, a town on the North Sea coast of Northeast England, in 1950. He has an elder sister, Madeleine, and a younger brother, Peter. His Parents were Cecile and Maurice Stack.

Father Michael was Ordained a Catholic Priest by Bishop Leo McCartie, also born in Hartlepool, in Lichfield, Staffordshire on July 18th, 1987 (Archdiocese of Birmingham).

Father Michael Stack is also the National Chaplain and Ecclesiastical Adviser for the Association of Catholic Nurses in England and Wales (www.catholicnurses.org.uk).

Over 20 years of Michael's Ministry has been in Health Care as a Hospital Chaplain:

- 1987-1990 New Cross Hospital, now part of the Royal Wolverhampton NHS Trust.
- 1990-1993 The Queen Elizabeth Hospital, now part of the University Hospitals Birmingham NHS Foundation Trust.
- 1990-1993 Birmingham Maternity Hospital, now part of Birmingham Women's and Children's NHS Foundation Trust.
- 1990-1993 The Queen Elizabeth Mental Health Unit, now part of Birmingham and Solihull Mental Health NHS Foundation Trust (BSMHFT).
- 1995-2000 George Eliot Hospital, now part of the George Eliot Hospital NHS Trust.
- 1995 Mary Ann Evans Hospice, Nuneaton.
- 2007-2016 University Hospitals Coventry & Warwickshire NHS Trust.
- 2007-2016 Hospital of St Cross Hospital, Rugby now part of the University Hospitals Coventry & Warwickshire NHS Trust.
- 2007-2016 Coventry Myton Hospice.
- 2018-2020 Semi-retirement within Christ the King Parish, Coventry.
- 2020-Present. Retired in East Anglia and helping at the local parishes in the area.